Blossoming Maternity

Essential Guide to a First Time Pregnancy

By

Dr. Faiz Ahmad

MBBS, MD

Table of Contents

About this book

"Blossoming Maternity: Essential Guide to a First-Time Pregnancy" is a comprehensive book particularly planned to help those who are going through their first pregnancy journey. This book is like a reliable friend that offers easy to understand information and advice about all the stages of pregnancy, from the moment you find out you are expecting to the moment when you meet your baby.

Inside this book, you will find guidance on understanding the changes happening in your body, how to eat well and stay active for a healthy pregnancy, and ways to manage the common discomforts that might come your way. It even covers important topics like choosing the right healthcare provider, planning for labor and delivery, and taking care of yourself after your baby arrives.

You will discover tips for creating a supportive environment, communicating with your partner, and preparing emotionally for the changes that come with motherhood. It is like having a helpful friend who answers your questions and offers a helping hand during this amazing journey.

"Blossoming Maternity" is here to make your first-time pregnancy experience smoother and more enjoyable. Whether you are curious about what to expect or need advice on taking care of yourself and your baby, this guide is by your side, offering information that is easy to understand and apply. Remember, every pregnancy is unique, but having a reliable resource like this book can make the journey more exciting and less overwhelming.

How to use this book

Using the book **"Blossoming Maternity: Your Essential Guide to a First-Time Pregnancy"** is like having a friendly and knowledgeable companion throughout your pregnancy journey.

Start from the Beginning: Begin by reading the introduction to understand what the book is all about. This part will get you excited about the journey you are about to embark on.

Take It Step by Step: The book is divided into chapters, each focusing on different aspects of pregnancy. You do not have to read it all in on go! Start with the chapters that interest you the most or the ones that are relevant to your current stag of pregnancy.

Read, Reflect, and Plan: As you read each chapter, take your time to absorb the information. Think about how it applies to your condition. Take notes or highlight important points if you want.

Follow the Checklists: The book includes checklists for pregnancy preparation, labor, and postpartum. These are like to-do lists that can help you stay organized and prepared. Follow them as you move along in your journey.

Use the Glossary: If you come across a word you are not familiar with, do not worry! The glossary at the end of the book will explain it in simple language.

Apply Practical Tips: Throughout the book, you'll find practical tips and advice. Consider how you can apply these suggestions to your own life. For example, if the book talks about eating well during pregnancy, think about incorporating nutritious foods into your meals.

Reflect on Your Feelings: Pregnancy can bring up a lot of emotions. Use the chapters that talk about emotional changes and stress management to reflect on your feelings and learn techniques to cope.

Discuss with Your Partner: If you have a partner, consider reading relevant sections together and discussing how you both feel about certain topics. This can strengthen your bond and help you navigate the journey together.

Seek Professional Help: While the book provides valuable information, remember that every pregnancy is unique. If you have specific concerns or questions, do not hesitate to visit healthcare professionals.

Celebrate Your Progress: As you move through the book and your pregnancy, celebrate your achievements and Milestones. Whether it is finishing a chapter or preparing for labor, every step is a part of your amazing journey.

Remember, this book is here to support you, not stress you out. Use it as a tool to gain knowledge, build confidence, and make your first-time pregnancy a beautiful and mem-orable experience.

Introduction

Welcome to the amazing world of pregnancy! A journey filled with inspiring moments, profound changes, and the miraculous creation of new life. In this introduction, we will delve into the fascinating miracle that is pregnancy, as well as explore the fundamental aspects that make it such a remarkable and transformative experience.

The Miracle of Pregnancy

Pregnancy is a natural and inspiring process that occurs within the female body. It is a time when a tiny, seemingly invisible cell begins to grow and develop into a fully-formed human being. From the moment of conception, a beautiful dance of biological events unfolds, leading to the birth of a precious baby. The sheer magic of this journey never fails to captivate and humble us as we witness the marvels of life coming into existence.

Understanding the Biological Process

At the heart of this fascinating journey lies the biological process of pregnancy. It all begins with the meeting of a sperm and an egg, which combine to form a zygote. This zygote then embarks on an extraordinary voyage of cell division and multiplication, gradually forming the embryo and eventually the fetus. Throughout the nine months of pregnancy, the mother's body undergoes numerous changes, adapting itself to nurture and protect the growing life within.

We will explore the fascinating stags of development that occur during pregnancy, from the early days of conception to the magical moment of birth. Understanding these stags will not only deepen your appreciation for the miracle of life but also equip you with valuable insights into the well-being of both the expectant mother and her precious baby.

Embracing the Journey of Motherhood

Pregnancy is not merely a biological process; it is a profound journey of motherhood. From the moment a woman learns she is pregnant, her life takes on a new and remarkable dimension. It is a time of emotional shifts, from excitement and joy to anxiety and anticipation. Throughout this voyage, a woman's heart opens up to the concept of nurturing and caring for a life beyond her own.

As the journey unfolds, we will explore the emotional and psychological aspects of becoming a mother, addressing the hopes and fears that may arise during this transformative period. We will discuss the significance of prenatal care, the support of loved ones, and the empowerment that comes with embracing the role of a mother.

In this guide, we aim to provide you with a comprehensive understanding of the miracle of pregnancy. Whether you are a expectant mother, a partner, a family member, or simply someone curious about the marvels of life, this book is designed to be your essential companion throughout this enchanting journey. So, let us embark together on this incredible adventure of blossoming maternity and celebrate the joy and wonder that pregnancy brings into our lives.

Chapter 1: Preparing for the Journey
Understanding Your Body

- **Menstrual Cycle and Ovulation**
- **Recognizing Fertile Days**

In this chapter, we will delve into the fascinating mechanisms of your body, particularly concerning the menstrual cycle and ovulation. Understanding these natural process is crucial, as they play a vital role in your journey toward motherhood. So, let's explore the complexities of your body and learn how to recognize your fertile days.

The Menstrual Cycle

The menstrual cycle is a remarkable and regular occurrence in the life of most women of reproductive age. It is a series of natural changes that happen in the body every month, preparing it for the possibility of pregnancy. The cycle usually lasts around 28 days, but it can vary from woman to woman.

We will break down the menstrual cycle into its key phases and explain what happens during each phase. From the shedding of the uterine lining during menstruation to the preparation of the uterus for potential pregnancy, we will provide you with a clear understanding of this fundamental process.

Ovulation - Your Fertile Window

Ovulation is a pivotal event in the menstrual cycle and is the key to conception. During ovulation, a mature egg is released from the ovary, making its way down the fallopian tube. If sperm is present in the fallopian tube at this time, fertilization may occur, lading to pregnancy. We will explore the signs and signals that indicate ovulation, helping you recognize your fertile days. Understanding when you are ovulating is essential if you are trying to conceive or even if you want to avoid pregnancy. We will also discuss the role of hormones in the ovulation process and how they influence your body throughout the menstrual cycle.

Recognizing Your Fertile Days

Knowing when you are fertile is crucial for anyone planning to start a family or trying to prevent pregnancy. We will introduce various methods to help you track and predict your fertile days.

Charting Basal Body Temperature (BBT): We will explain how your body temperature changes subtly during the menstrual cycle and how charting your BBT can indicate when ovulation is likely to occur.

Charting basal body temperature (BBT) is a valuable method for detecting ovulation and understanding your menstrual cycle.

How you can do it

Step 1: Get Prepared

- You will need a basal body thermometer, which is more sensitive than a regular thermometer.
- You can find them at most drugstores or online.
- Keep your thermometer and a notebook or a fertility tracking app beside your bed.

Step 2: Timing is everything

- Start taking your temperature every morning as soon as you wake up, before you even get out of bed.
- Try to take your temperature at the same time every day, as consistency is important for accurate results.
- It's best to start tracking your temperature from the beginning of your menstrual cycle (the first day of your period).

Step 3: Recording the Temperature

- Use the basal body thermometer to take your temperature orally, vaginally, or rectally.
- Choose one method and stick with it for consistent results.
- Record your temperature in your notebook or fertility app every day.

- Make a simple line graph with the dates on the bottom and temperatures on the side.

Step 4: Observe the Pattern

- In the first half of your menstrual cycle, your temperatures will generally be lower.
- After ovulation, due to hormonal changes, your BBT will rise and stay elevated until your next period.
- You are looking for a clear temperature shift – usually about 0. 5 to 1. 0 degree Fahrenheit (0. 3 to 0. 6 degrees Celsius) higher than the temperatures before ovulation.

Step 5: Identifying Ovulation

- Ovulation typically occurs on the day of the temperature shift or the day after.
- After a few cycles of charting, you might notice a pattern of when ovulation usually happens for you.
- You're most fertile a day or two before the temperature rise, so this is a good time for trying to conceive if that's your goal.

Step 6: Other Signs and Considerations

- Remember that BBT alone is not foolproof for predicting ovulation.

- You can also pay attention to cervical mucus changes and other fertility signs.
- Illness, poor sleep, alcohol, and certain medications can influence your BBT, so keep these factors in mind.

Step 7: Be Patient and Consistent

- Charting BBT requires patience, as it may take a few cycles to understand your unique pattern.
- Consistency in taking your temperature at the same time each day is crucial for accurate results.

Remember, while BBT charting can provide insights into your menstrual cycle and ovulation, it might not work for everyone. If you have irregular periods or suspect fertility issues, it is a good idea to consult a healthcare professional.

Monitoring Cervical Mucus: Your cervical mucus changes in consistency throughout the menstrual cycle. We will guide you on how to observe and interpret these changes to identify fertile days.

Ovulation Predictor Kits (OPKs): These kits are designed to predict ovulation by detecting certain hormones in your urine. We will explain how to use them effectively to pin-point your fertile window.

By the end of this chapter, you will have a deeper un-der-standing of the intricate processes at play within your body. You will be better equipped to identify your fertile days accurately, whether you are trying to conceive or practicing natural birth control methods. Understanding your body is an empowering step to-ward embracing your fertility and making informed choices on your journey toward motherhood.

Nutrition and Exercise

- **Creating a Balanced Diet for Pregnancy**
- **Safe and Recommended Exercises**

Welcome to the chapter on Nutrition and Exercise during pregnancy, where we will explore the essential aspects of maintaining a healthy lifestyle for both you and your growing baby. Taking care of your body through a balanced diet and safe exercises is crucial in ensuring a smooth and fulfilling journey to motherhood.

Creating a Balanced Diet for Pregnancy

Eating well during pregnancy is one of the best ways to support your baby's growth and keep yourself healthy. We will guide you in creating a balanced diet that provides all the necessary nutrients for you and your little one.

a) The Power of Nutrient-Rich Foods

Pregnancy is a special time when your body needs extra nutrients to support both your health and the growth of your baby. Nutrient rich foods are like the superhero team that ensures a healthy pregnancy journey. Here is why they are so powerful

1. Baby's Growth and Development

Nutrient-rich foods are packed with vitamins, minerals, and proteins that fuel your baby's growth and development. These nutrients help build tiny organs, bonds, and brain cells, giving your baby a strong start in life.

2. Mom's Well-being

Eating well balanced, nutrient-rich foods can help prevent pregnancy discomforts like fatigue and morning sickness. They also provide energy to keep you feeling good and support your body's changes.

3. Building Immunity

Nutrient-rich foods contain antioxidants that strengthen your immune system. This shield helps protect you and your baby from illnesses during this crucial time.

4. Avoiding Nutrient Deficiencies

Curtain nutrients, like folic acid and iron, are extra important during pregnancy. Nutrient-rich foods help you avoid deficiencies that can affect your baby's health.

5. Healthy Wight Gain

Eating nutrient-rich foods helps you gain a healthy amount of weight during pregnancy. This supports your baby's growth without causing excess weight gain, which can lead to complications.

Top Nutrient-Rich Foods for Pregnancy

Fruits and Vegetables: Packed with vitamins, minerals, and fiber. Go for a colorful variety.

Lean Proteins: Chicken, fish, beans, and lentils provide essential amino acids for growth.

Whole Grains: Brown rice, whole what bread, and oats offer sustained energy?

Dairy Products: Milk, yogurt, and cheese are rich in calcium and vitamin D for strong bones.

Healthy Fats: Avocado, nuts, and seeds are sources of essential fatty acids.

b) Folic Acid and Iron: These two essential nutrients play a vital role in preventing birth defects and supporting your baby's development.

c) Calcium for Strong Bones: Calcium is crucial for the de-velopment of your baby's bones and teeth

d) Omega-3 Fatty Acids: Omega-3s are essential for the healthy development of your baby's brain and eyes.

e) Hydration: Staying hydrated is vital during pregnancy.

Safe and Recommended Exercises

Exercise can bring numerous benefits during pregnancy, such as improving your mood, boosting energy levels, and promoting better sleep. However, safety is of utmost importance, and certain exercises may need to be modified or avoided altogether. We will guide you through safe and recommended exercises for expectant mothers.

a) Prenatal Yoga: Yoga is an excellent way to enhance flexibility and strength while also promoting relaxation and stress relief.

b) Walking: Taking brisk walks is a low impact exercise that is gentle on your body while still providing cardiovascular benefits.

c) Swimming: Swimming is a wonderful full body workout that helps to alleviate pressure on joints and ligaments.

d) Pelvic Floor Exercises: Strengthening your pelvic floor muscles can be beneficial during pregnancy and postpartum. We will explain how to perform these exercises correctly.

e) Avoiding High-Risk Activities: Certain activities, such as contact sports or exercises with a risk of falling, should be avoided during pregnancy to ensure the safety of both you and your baby.

Throughout this chapter, we will emphasize the importance of listening to your body and consulting with your healthcare provider before starting or continuing any exercise routine. Additionally, we will provide tips on staying motivated and making exercise a fun and enjoyable part of your pregnancy journey.

Remember, taking care of yourself through a balanced diet and safe exercises will not only benefit you but also contribute to the healthy development of your precious baby. Embrace this opportunity to nourish your body and cultivate a positive and active lifestyle during this extraordinary time of blossoming maternity.

Lifestyle Changes

- **The Importance of Avoiding Harmful Substances**
- **Stress Management and Relaxation Techniques**

Congratulations on your pregnancy! In this chapter, we will discuss essential lifestyle changes that will contribute to a healthy and happy pregnancy. Making positive choices during this special time will not only benefit you but also sup-port the wellbeing of your growing baby.

The Importance of Avoiding Harmful Substances

During pregnancy, it's crucial to be mindful of what you put into your body, as it directly affects your baby's development. Let's explore the harmful substances that should be avoided during pregnancy

a) Smoking and Second hand Smoke

Smoking is harmful to both you and your baby, as it reduces the oxygen supply to the baby and can lead to various complications. Additionally, exposure to secondhand smoke can also be harmful. Quitting smoking or avoiding places where smoking occurs is vital for a healthy pregnancy.

b) Alcohol

Alcohol can have severe consequences for your baby's development, leading to fetal alcohol spectrum disorders. It's best to avoid alcohol entirely during pregnancy.

c) Illicit Drugs and Medications

Using illegal drugs or certain medications during pregnancy can harm your baby. Always consult with your healthcare provider before taking any medications, including over-the-counter drugs, to ensure they are safe for pregnancy.

d) Caffeine

While moderate caffeine intake is generally considered safe during pregnancy, excessive caffeine consumption should be avoided. Stick to the recommended limit of 200-300 mg per day, equivalent to about one 12-ounce cup of coffee.

Stress Management and Relaxation Techniques

Pregnancy can bring various emotions and challenges, and managing stress is essential for your well-being and the health of your baby. Let's explore some relaxation techniques to help you stay calm and centered

a) Deep Breathing

Practice deep breathing exercises to relax your mind and body. Take slow, deep breaths, and focus on each breath as it enters and laves your body.

b) Gentle Exercise

Engage in gentle exercises like prenatal yoga or walking to release tension and boost your mood. Always consult your healthcare provider before starting any new exercise routine.

c) Rest and Sleep

Adequate rest is crucial during pregnancy. Ensure you get enough sleep each night, and listen to your body when it needs extra rest during the day.

d) Meditation and Mindfulness

Practicing meditation and mindfulness can help you stay present and reduce anxiety. Find a quiet space, close your eyes, and focus on the present moment.

e) Support System

Share your flings and concerns with your partner, family, or friends. Having a support system can provide comfort and encouragement throughout your pregnancy journey.

By making these lifestyle changes and taking care of yourself, you are providing the best possible environment for your baby's growth and development. Embrace this transformative time with positivity and love, and remember to seek guidance from your healthcare provider if you have any questions or concerns. Wishing you a joyful and healthy pregnancy journey!

Discussing Parenthood

- **Communicating with Your Partner**
- **Preparing for Emotional Changes**

Communicating with Your Partner

Parenthood is a joint venture, and discussing your thoughts and feelings with your partner is crucial. Let's delve into effective communication strategies to strengthen your bond during this exciting time:

a) Share Your Hopes and Dreams

Take the time to express your hopes and dreams about becoming parents. Discuss the kind of parents you aspire to be and the values you want to instill in your child. This will help create a shared vision for your family's future.

b) Address Fears and Concerns

It's normal to have fears and concerns about parenthood. Create a safe space where you both can openly talk about any worries or anxieties you may have. Supporting each other through honest conversations will help alleviate fears and foster understanding.

c) Division of Responsibilities

Discuss how you plan to divide responsibilities when the baby arrives. Having clarity on roles and expectations can prevent misunderstandings and ensure a harmonious partnership in parenting.

d) Attend Prenatal Classes Together

Consider attending prenatal classes together. These classes offer valuable insights into pregnancy, childbirth, and newborn care, and they provide an excellent opportunity to bond as a couple.

Preparing for Emotional Changes

Becoming a parent is a profound emotional journey that brings a mix of joy, excitement, and, at times, uncertainty. Let's explore how to prepare for these emotional changes:

a) Embrace the Rollercoaster of Emotions

It's normal to experience a range of emotions during pregnancy and after childbirth. From elation to occasional feelings of overwhelm, allow yourself to feel all emotions without judgment.

b) Seek Emotional Support

Rely on your partner, friends, and family for emotional support. Having a strong support system can make the journey to parenthood feel less daunting.

c) Take Time for Self-Care

Prioritize self-care to nurture your emotional well-being. Engage in activities that bring you joy and relaxation, whether it's reading, spending time in nature, or practicing mindfulness.

d) Learn about Postpartum Emotions

Educate yourselves about postpartum emotions, commonly known as the "baby blues." Knowing what to expect can help both you and your partner navigate this phase with compassion and understanding.

By communicating openly with your partner and preparing for emotional changes together, you are strengthening your connection as a team. Remember, parenthood is a journey of growth, love, and shared experiences. Embrace this transformative time with open hearts, and know that you have each other's unwavering support. Wishing you a beautiful and fulfilling journey into parenthood!

Chapter 2: Conception and Early Signs of Pregnancy

Understanding Conception
(The Journey to New Life)

- **How Fertilization Occurs**
- **Identifying the Best Time to Conceive**

Welcome to the chapter on Understanding Conception! In this chapter, we will take a fascinating journey into the world of fertilization and explore how you can identify the best time to conceive. Conception is the magical moment when new life begins, and understanding this process can be an essential step on your path to parenthood.

How Fertilization Occurs

Fertilization is the remarkable process where a sperm cell meets an egg cell, resulting in the creation of a zygote - the first stage of your baby's life. Let's dive into the steps of fertilization:

a) The Journey of Sperm

When a man ejaculates, millions of tiny sperm are released into the woman's vagina. These sperm start a challenging and exciting journey, swimming through the cervix, up the uterus, and into the fallopian tubes.

b) Meeting the Egg

For fertilization to occur, a sperm must successfully find and penetrate the egg in the fallopian tube. This incredible event is known as conception and happens within a day or two after ovulation.

c) The Zygote

Once a sperm successfully enters the egg, they merge to form a zygote - the very beginning of your baby's develop-ment. The zygote begins to divide and grow as it travels down the fallopian tube towards the uterus.

Identifying the Best Tim to Conceive

Knowing when you are most fertile can significantly in-crease your chances of conceiving. Let's explore how to identify the best time for conception

a) Tracking Your Menstrual Cycle

Understanding your menstrual cycle is essential in deter-mining your fertile days. Typically, ovulation occurs around the middle of your cycle, approximately 14 days before the start of your next period.

b) Recognizing Ovulation Signs

During ovulation, your body may show certain signs, such as a change in cervical mucus (it becomes clear, slippery, and stretchy) and a slight increase in basal body tempera-ture. Paying attention to these signs can help you predict when you are most likely to ovulate.

c) Ovulation Predictor Kits (OPKs)

Using ovulation predictor kits is another helpful method. These kits detect hormone levels in your urine, indicating when ovulation is approaching.

d) Fertility Apps and Charts

Fertility apps and charting can be valuable tools for tracking your menstrual cycle and identifying your fertile days. They can help you record ovulation signs and predict your most fertile window.

By understanding how fertilization occurs and identifying your most fertile days, you are empowering yourself with knowledge to plan for conception. Remember that each person's body is unique, and it may take time to conceive. Be patient, stay positive, and remember that your journey to parenthood is a beautiful and miraculous process. Best of luck on your exciting path ahead!

Recognizing Early Pregnancy Symptoms
(A Journey of Transformations)

- **Common Physical Changes**
- **Emotional and Psychological Changes**

Welcome to the chapter dedicated to Recognizing Early Pregnancy Symptoms! In this chapter, we will explore the various physical, emotional, and psychological changes that may indicate the exciting beginning of your pregnancy. Each woman's experience is unique, but understanding these early signs can help you recognize the miraculous journey of motherhood unfolding within you.

Common Physical Changes

During the early stages of pregnancy, your body undergoes remarkable transformations as it prepares to nurture a growing life.

Let's delve into some common physical changes that you may experience:

a) Missed Period:

A missed menstrual period is often the first sign that you might be pregnant. However, some women may experience light bleeding or spotting during early pregnancy, often referred to as implantation bleeding.

b) Tender and Swollen Breasts:

Your breasts may feel tender and appear swollen due to the hormonal changes happening in your body. You may also notice that your nipples become more sensitive.

c) Fatigue:

Feeling more tired than usual is a common early pregnancy symptom. Your body is working hard to support the pregnancy, which can leave you feeling fatigued.

d) Nausea and Morning Sickness:

Morning sickness, which can occur at any time of the day, may make you feel nauseous and may even lead to vomiting. This is caused by the rise in pregnancy hormones.

e) Frequent Urination:

You may find yourself visiting the bathroom more frequently than before due to hormonal changes and increased blood flow to your pelvic region.

Emotional and Psychological Changes:

Pregnancy brings about a range of emotions as you embark on this life-changing journey. Let's explore some common emotional and psychological changes during early pregnancy:

a) Mood Swings

Fluctuating hormones can lead to mood swings, causing you to feel elated one moment and tearful the next. These emotional changes are entirely normal during pregnancy.

b) Heightened Emotions

You may find yourself experiencing heightened emotions, feeling more sensitive, or being more easily moved by things.

c) Anxiety and Excitement

Feeling anxious and excited about the prospect of becoming a parent is entirely normal. The anticipation of this new chapter in your life can bring a mix of emotions.

d) Changes in Appetite

You may notice changes in your appetite, ranging from increased cravings to aversions to certain foods. These changes are influenced by hormonal shifts.

It's important to remember that every pregnancy is different, and not all women experience the same symptoms. Some may have several early pregnancy signs, while others may have only a few or none at all. If you suspect you might be pregnant or are experiencing any of these early symptoms, consider taking a home pregnancy test or consult with your healthcare provider for confirmation.

Embrace this incredible time of transformation and trust in your body's ability to nurture new life. Allow yourself to experience the joy and wonder of pregnancy as you embark on this beautiful journey to motherhood. Congratulations on this exciting phase of your life!

Confirming Pregnancy
(From Home Tests to Professional Verification)

- **Home Pregnancy Tests**
- **Visiting a Healthcare Provider**

Welcome to the chapter on Confirming Pregnancy! In this chapter, we will explore the different methods you can use to confirm whether you are pregnant. From the convenience of home pregnancy tests to the expertise of healthcare providers, we will guide you through the process of obtaining accurate and reliable results.

Home Pregnancy Tests

Home pregnancy tests are a quick and accessible way to find out if you are pregnant. These tests work by detecting a hormone called human chorionic gonadotropin (hCG) in your urine. Let's explore how to use home pregnancy tests effectively:

a) Timing Matters

For the most accurate results, it's essential to take the test at the right time. Most home pregnancy tests can detect hCG in your urine about a wk. after your missed period. However, some tests claim to offer results even earlier.

b) Read the Instructions

Each home pregnancy test comes with clear instructions on how to use it correctly. It's crucial to read and follow the instructions carefully to ensure accurate results.

c) Collect a Sample

Collect a sample of your urine in a clean, dry container as per the instructions. Some tests require you to urinate directly on the test stick.

d) Wait for the Results

After taking the test, you will need to wait for a few minutes for the results to appear. A positive result typically shows as two lines or a plus sign, while a negative result is indicated by a single line or a minus sign.

e) Consider Taking a Second Test

If you get a negative result but still suspect you might be pregnant or your period doesn't arrive, consider taking another test a few days later or visit a healthcare provider for further evaluation.

Visiting a Healthcare Provider

For a definitive confirmation of pregnancy and personalized care, visiting a healthcare provider is the next step. Here's what to expect during your visit:

a) Professional Pregnancy Test

Healthcare providers can perform a pregnancy test similar to the home tests, but with medical-grade accuracy.

b) Blood Test and Urinalysis

In some cases, your healthcare provider may order a blood test to measure the levels of hCG in your blood or perform a urinalysis to confirm pregnancy.

c) Initial Consultation

During your visit, your healthcare provider will discuss your medical history, review any symptoms you may have, and provide information about prenatal care and what to expect during your pregnancy.

d) Pregnancy Confirmation

After obtaining the test results, your healthcare provider will confirm whether you are pregnant and estimate your due date based on the first day of your last menstrual period.

Visiting a healthcare provider is an excellent opportunity to address any questions or concerns you may have and receive guidance on how to maintain a healthy pregnancy. Regular prenatal care is essential for monitoring the well-being of both you and your baby throughout your pregnancy journey.

Remember, confirming your pregnancy is an exciting and significant moment. Whether you choose to start with a home pregnancy test or visit a healthcare provider right away, the confirmation of new life is a special time filled with hope and anticipation. Congratulations on this remarkable milestone in your journey to motherhood!

Chapter 3: Navigating the First Trimester
Prenatal Care
(Nurturing a Healthy Pregnancy)

- **Choosing a Healthcare Provider**
- **The Importance of Regular Check-ups**

Welcome to the chapter on Prenatal Care! In this chapter, we will explore the essential aspects of caring for yourself and your baby during pregnancy. From choosing a healthcare provider to the importance of regular check-ups, prenatal care is a crucial foundation for a healthy and happy pregnancy journey.

Choosing a Healthcare Provider

Selecting the right healthcare provider is an important decision that will shape your prenatal care experience. Here's how to make an informed choice:

a) Obstetrician-Gynecologist (OB-GYN)

An OB-GYN is a medical doctor specializing in women's reproductive health. They are trained to provide compre-hensive prenatal care, including de-livery, if you plan to give birth in a hospital.

b) Certified Nurse-Midwife (CNM)

A CNM is a registered nurse with advanced training in midwifery and prenatal care. They focus on supporting natural births and can also provide care in birthing cantors or hospitals.

c) Family Practitioner

Some family practitioners have experience in prenatal care and may be an option for women with low-risk pregnancies.

Consider factors such as the provider's experience, location, and philosophy of care when making your decision. It's essential to feel comfortable and confident in the care you will receive throughout your pregnancy.

The Importance of Regular Check-ups

Regular prenatal check-ups are essential to monitor the health of both you and your baby. Let's explore the significance of these appointments:

a) Early Prenatal Visits

Your first prenatal visit typically occurs around 8 to 12 weeks of pregnancy. During this visit, your healthcare provider will review your medical history, conduct a physical examination, and order initial tests to confirm your pregnancy and assess your overall health.

b) Monitoring Baby's Growth and Development

Throughout your pregnancy, you will have regular check-ups to monitor your baby's growth and development. Your healthcare provider will perform routine tests, such as ultra-sounds and blood tests, to ensure your baby is thriving.

c) Managing Health Conditions:

If you have any pre-existing health conditions, such as diabetes or high blood pressure, prenatal visits are crucial for managing these conditions during pregnancy.

d) Addressing Concerns and Questions:

Prenatal check-ups offer an opportunity to address any concerns or questions you may have. Your healthcare provider is there to offer guidance, support, and information throughout your pregnancy journey.

e) Preparing for Labor and Delivery

As your due date approaches, prenatal visits will focus on preparing for labor and delivery. Your healthcare provider will discuss birth plans, pain management options, and what to expect during delivery.

Regular prenatal check-ups ensure that any potential issues or complications are detected early, allowing for prompt intervention and optimal care for you and your baby.

Remember, prenatal care is a partnership between you and your healthcare provider. Engaging in open communication and following their guidance will contribute to a healthy and safe pregnancy. Embrace each prenatal visit as an opportunity to celebrate the growth of your baby and nurture the bond between you and your little one. Congratulations on taking this important step in caring for yourself and your baby during this remarkable journey of motherhood!

Coping with Morning Sickness
(Navigating Nausea with Confidence)

- **Tips and Remedies for Nausea**
- **When to Seek Medical Advice**

Welcome to the chapter dedicated to Coping with Morning Sickness! In this chapter, we will explore practical tips and remedies to help you manage the common discomfort of nausea during pregnancy. Additionally, we will discuss when it is appropriate to seek medical advice for morning sickness symptoms.

Tips and Remedies for Nausea

Morning sickness, which can occur at any time of the day, is a common pregnancy symptom experienced by many ex-pectant mothers. Her are some tips and remedies to ease the discomfort:

a) Small, Frequent Meals

Eating small, frequent meals throughout the day can help stabilize blood sugar levels and reduce feelings of nausea.

b) *Avoiding Trigger Foods*

Identify foods or smells that trigger your nausea and try to avoid them. Common triggers include strong odors and greasy or spicy foods.

c) Stay Hydrated

Drink plenty of fluids, especially water, to stay hydrated. Sip fluids slowly rather than gulping large amounts at once.

d) Ginger

Ginger has natural anti-nausea properties. Try sipping ginger tea, eating ginger candies, or using ginger in your meals to alleviate nausea.

e) Fresh Air

Spending time outdoors or in well-ventilated spaces can help reduce feelings of nausea.

f) Acupressure

Some women find relief from morning sickness by using acupressure wristbands, which apply gentle pressure to specific points on the wrist.

g) Rest and Relaxation

Make sure you get enough rest and practice relaxation techniques to reduce stress, which can contribute to feelings of nausea.

When to Seek Medical Advice

In most cases, morning sickness is a normal part of pregnancy and does not pose a significant health risk to you or your baby. However, there are instances when seeking medical advice is essential:

a) Severe or Persistent Nausea

If your nausea is severe, persistent, or accompanied by vomiting excessively, it's crucial to consult your healthcare provider. Severe morning sickness, known as hyperemesis gravidarum, may require medical intervention.

b) Dehydration

If you are unable to keep fluids down or notice signs of dehydration, such as dark urine or extreme thirst, seek medical attention promptly.

c) Weight Loss

Significant weight loss during pregnancy due to nausea and vomiting requires medical evaluation.

d) Urinary Tract Infections (UTIs)

Frequent vomiting can increase the risk of UTIs. If you experience symptoms like pain or burning during urination, consult your healthcare provider.

e) High Fever or Abdominal Pain

If you develop a high fever or experience severe abdominal pain along with morning sickness, seek medical attention immediately.

Remember, morning sickness is a temporary phase of pregnancy for most women, and it usually improves as the pregnancy progresses. If you have any concerns about your morning sickness symptoms or are unsure whether they are within the normal rang, don't hesitate to reach out to your healthcare provider. Their guidance and support will help you navigate morning sickness with confidence and ensure a healthy and comfortable pregnancy journey. Congratulations on this exciting time of your life!

Understanding the Changes in Your Body
(Embracing the Journey of Transformation)

- **Hormonal and Physical Changes**
- **Common Discomforts and How to Manage**

Welcome to the chapter dedicated to Understanding the Changes in Your Body during pregnancy! In this chapter, we will explore the incredible hormonal and physical changes that occur within you as you embark on this miraculous journey of motherhood. We will also address common discomforts that may arise and provide practical tips on how to manage them with ease.

Hormonal and Physical Changes

Pregnancy triggers a cascade of hormonal changes that support the growth and development of your baby. Let's delve into some of the remarkable hormonal and physical changes you may experience:

a) Increased Levels of Hormones

During pregnancy, your body produces higher levels of hormones like estrogen and progesterone, which play a vital role in nurturing your baby and preparing your body for childbirth.

b) Growth of the Uterus

As your baby grows, so does your uterus. It expands to ac-commodate the developing fetus, gradually pushing your abdominal organs to make room for the growing life inside you.

c) Breast Changes

Your breasts undergo significant changes, becoming larger and more sensitive. These changes are in preparation for breastfeeding after your baby is born.

d) Weight Gain

Wight gain is a natural part of pregnancy and is necessary for your baby's healthy development. Your healthcare pro-vider will monitor your weight gain to ensure it falls within a healthy rang.

e) Stretch Marks

Due to the rapid stretching of the skin, you may develop stretch marks on your abdomen, breasts, and thighs. This marks are entirely normal and often fade with time.

Common Discomforts and How to Manage Them

While pregnancy is a beautiful journey, it may also bring about some common discomforts. Let's explore these discomforts and discover effective ways to manage them:

a) Nausea and Morning Sickness

Try eating small, frequent meals and avoid trigger foods. Ginger and relaxation techniques can also help alleviate nausea.

b) Fatigue

Listen to your body and prioritize rest. Take short naps and ensure you get enough sleep at night.

c) Backache and Joint Pain

Practice good posture and avoid heavy lifting. Gentle exercises like prenatal yoga can strengthen your back and alleviate joint pain.

d) Heartburn

Eat smaller meals and avoid spicy or acidic foods. Elevating your upper body while sleeping can also help reduce heartburn.

e) Swollen Feet and Ankles

Elevate your legs whenever possible and wear comfortable, supportive shoes. Avoid standing for prolonged periods.

f) Constipation

Stay hydrated, eat fiber-rich foods, and engage in regular physical activity to promote healthy digestion.

Remember, every woman's pregnancy journey is unique, and the changes in your body may vary. . Embrace these changes with an open heart, knowing that they are part of the miraculous process of nurturing new life within you. If you experience any discomforts that are persistent or concerning, don't hesitate to discuss them with your healthcare provider. Their guidance and support will ensure you have a healthy and enjoyable pregnancy experience. Congratulations on embracing the wonderful transformations taking place within you!

Creating a Supportive Environment
(Embracing the Journey with Loved Ones)

- **Sharing the News with Family and Friends**
- **Joining Support Groups and Online Communities**

Welcome to the chapter dedicated to Creating a Supportive Environment during your pregnancy! In this chapter, we will explore the importance of sharing the exciting news with family and friends, as well as the benefits of joining support groups and online communities. Building a strong support system will help you feel nurtured and cherished as you embark on this amazing journey of motherhood.

Sharing the News with Family and Friends

Announcing your pregnancy to your loved ones can be a heartwarming and joyous experience. Here are some tips for sharing the news

a) Choose the Right Time

Take your time to decide when and how you want to share the news. Some couples prefer to wait until after the first trimester, while others can't wait to share their happiness right away.

b) Make it Special

Consider making the announcement memorable. You can plan a special gathering, give personalized gifts, or involve older siblings if you already have children.

c) Embrace Different Reactions

Remember that everyone may react differently to the news. Some may be overjoyed, while others might need time to process the information. Embrace their responses with un-derstanding and love.

d) Seek Support and Advice

Your family and friends can be a great source of support and advice during your pregnancy journey. Don't hesitate to lean on them for encouragement and guid-ance.

Joining Support Groups and Online Communities

Connecting with other expectant mothers and parents-to-be can be incredibly beneficial. Here's why joining support groups and online communities can enhance your pregnancy experience:

a) Shared Experiences

In these groups, you'll find individuals going through similar experiences, which can create a sense of camaraderie and understanding.

b) Access to Information

Support groups and online communities are a wealth of information. You can ask questions, share concerns, and learn from the experiences of others.

c) Emotional Support

Pregnancy can bring a range of emotions. Having a supportive community to share your feelings with can be comforting and reassuring.

d) Non-Judgmental Space

These groups offer a non-judgmental space where you can freely express your thoughts and concerns without fear of criticism.

e) Celebrate Milestones Together

As you reach different milestones during your pregnancy, you can celebrate them with others who understand the significance and excitement.

f) Postpartum Support

Many support groups extend their support beyond pregnancy, providing valuable resources for new parents navigating the postpartum period.

Remember, building a supportive environment during your pregnancy is not only essential for your well-being but also enhances your baby's development. Surrounding yourself with love, encouragement, and understanding contributes to a positive and fulfilling pregnancy experience. Whether it's the support of your family and friends or a support group or online community, embracing this journey with loved ones by your side will make it all the more meaningful and memorable. Congratulations on this special time in your life!

Chapter 4: The Second Trimester: Blossoming and Bonding

Embracing the Second Trimester
(A Time of Growth and Celebration)

- **Changes in the Baby's Development**
- **Celebrating Your Pregnancy**

Welcome to the chapter dedicated to Embracing the Second Trimester of your pregnancy! In this chapter, we will explore the exciting changes in your baby's development during this stage and the joy of celebrating this special time in your life.

Changes in the Baby's Development

The second trimester is a remarkable time when your baby undergoes significant growth and development. Let's delve into some of the exciting changes happening in your little one:

a) Rapid Growth

During the second trimester, your baby experiences a growth spurt. They go from being the size of a peach to reaching the length of a banana.

b) Developing Senses

Your baby's senses start to develop, and they can now taste, touch, and even hear sounds from the outside world, including your voice.

c) Movement and Kicks As your baby's muscles become stronger, you'll start to feel those precious little kicks and movements,

creating a beautiful bond between you and your baby.

d) Facial Features

Your baby's facial features become more defined, and tiny eyebrows, eyelashes, and lips begin to take shape.

e) Gender Reveal

For those who want to know the gender of their baby, the second trimester is usually the time when it becomes visible on an ultrasound.

Celebrating Your Pregnancy

The second trimester is often referred to as the "golden period" of pregnancy. With morning sickness typically subsiding and your energy levels returning, it's an excellent time to celebrate and cherish this special phase of your life:

a) Pregnancy Photoshoot

Consider having a pregnancy photoshoot to capture the beauty of this momentous time. You'll have lovely memories to cherish for years to come.

b) Baby Shower

A baby shower is a wonderful way for family and friends to come together and celebrate your impending arrival. It's a chance to receive well-wishes, gifts, and support.

c) Bonding with Your Partner

Embrace this time to bond with your partner, as you both prepare to welcome your baby into the world. Spend quality time together and talk about your dreams and aspirations for your growing family.

d) Pregnancy Journal

Keep a pregnancy journal to jot down your thoughts, feelings, and experiences throughout this trimester. It's a beautiful keepsake to reflect on in the future.

e) Preparing the Nursery

Consider starting to prepare the nursery for your baby's ar-rival. Choosing colors, decorating, and setting up the space can be an exciting and joyful process.

Remember, the second trimester is a precious time filled with anticipation and excitement. Embrace the changes happening in your baby's development and savor the special moments with your loved ones. Celebrating your pregnancy helps create cherished memories that will remain in your heart forever. Congratulations on reaching this significant milestone in your pregnancy journey!

Prenatal Tests and Ultrasounds
(Nurturing Your Baby's Health and Connection)

- **Understanding the Purpose of Tests**
- **Bonding with Your Baby through Ultrasound**

Welcome to the chapter dedicated to Prenatal Tests and Ultrasounds! In this chapter, we will explore the importance of prenatal tests and ultrasounds in ensuring your baby's health and well-being. Additionally, we'll discuss how ultrasounds provide a unique opportunity for you to bond with your little one even before they enter the world.

Understanding the Purpose of Tests

Prenatal tests play a vital role in monitoring your baby's development and identifying any potential health concerns. Let's explore the different types of prenatal tests and their purposes:

a) Blood Tests

Blood tests, such as the complete blood count (CBC) and blood glucose test, help assess your overall health and detect conditions like anemia and gestational diabetes.

b) Genetic Screening Tests

Genetic screening tests, like the first-trimester screening and cell-free DNA test, can provide information about the risk of certain genetic conditions in your baby.

c) Anatomy Ultrasound

The anatomy ultrasound, usually performed around 18-20 weeks, evaluates your baby's major organs and structures to ensure they are developing correctly.

d) Group B Streptococcus (GBS) Test

This test, performed later in pregnancy, checks for the presence of Group B streptococcus bacteria, which can be harmful to the baby during childbirth.

e) Glucose Tolerance Test

The glucose tolerance test helps identify gestational diabetes, a temporary form of diabetes that can develop during pregnancy.

Bonding with Your Baby through Ultrasound

Ultrasound scans offer an extraordinary opportunity for you to connect with your baby and witness their growth and movements. Here's how ultrasounds contribute to the bonding experience:

a) Seeing Your Baby's Features

Ultrasounds allow you to see your baby's face, hands, and feet. This visual connection can deepen the emotional bond you share with your little one.

b) Hearing Your Baby's Heartbeat

Listening to your baby's heartbeat during an ultrasound can be a heartwarming experience, reaffirming the miracle of life growing within you.

c) Watching Baby's Movements

As your baby moves and stretches in the womb, you can witness these delightful moments during an ultrasound, further connecting you with their presence.

d) Involving Your Partner

Ultrasounds are an excellent opportunity for your partner to bond with the baby as well. It's a shared experience that strengthens your connection as a family.

e) Early Gender Reveal

If you choose to find out your baby's gender, the ultrasound can provide a delightful early gender reveal, making the experience even more special.

Remember, prenatal tests and ultrasounds are essential for ensuring the health and well-being of both you and your baby. Embrace these opportunities to bond with your little one, fostering a loving connection before they arrive in your arms. Celebrate each milestone of your baby's development, knowing that these precious moments are the foundation of the loving relationship you'll share with your child throughout life. Congratulations on nurturing your baby's health and forging a beautiful connection even before birth!

Maintaining a Healthy Lifestyle
(Nurturing Your Body and Mind)

- **Exercise and Nutrition during the Second Trimester**
- **Sleep and Rest for Expectant Mothers**

Welcome to the chapter dedicated to Maintaining a Healthy Lifestyle during the second trimester of your pregnancy! In this chapter, we will explore the significance of exercise, nutrition, sleep, and rest in ensuring the well-being of both you and your baby. Implementation a healthy lifestyle during this phase will contribute to a happy and fulfilling pregnant-cy journey.

Exercise and Nutrition during the Second Trimester

Staying active and nourishing your body with the right foods are vital components of a healthy pregnancy. Let's delve into the benefits of exercise and nutrition during the second trimester

a) Exercise

Regular physical activity during pregnancy can improve your mood, boost energy levels, and promote better sleep. Safe and recommended exercises for the second trimester include walking, swimming, prenatal yoga, and low-impact aerobics. Consult your healthcare provider before starting any new exercise routine.

b) Proper Nutrition

A balanced diet rich in essential nutrients is essential for your baby's growth and development. Focus on eating a variety of fruits, vegetables, whole grains, lean proteins, and dairy products. Stay hydrated by drinking plenty of water throughout the day.

c) Wight Gain

During the second trimester, you will likely experience weight gain as your baby grows. Monitor your weight gain as per your healthcare provider's guidance to ensure it falls within a healthy range.

d) Managing Food Cravings

While it's okay to indulge in occasional cravings, try to maintain a balanced diet overall. Substitute healthier alternatives for unhealthy cravings to ensure you and your baby get the necessary nutrients.

Sleep and Rest for Expectant Mothers

Adequate sleep and rest are crucial for your well-being and your baby's development. Here's why getting enough rest during the second trimester is vital:

a) Enhancing Energy Levels

As your body works hard to support your baby's growth, sufficient rest can help replenish your energy levels.

b) Relieving Discomfort

Finding comfortable sleeping positions can help relieve common discomforts like backaches and heartburn.

c) Promoting Baby's Development

Rest is essential for your baby's development, as their body and brain continue to grow rapidly during the second trimester.

d) Stress Reduction

Ample rest can reduce stress and anxiety, contributing to a positive pregnancy experience.

e) Sleep Quality

Practice good sleep hygiene by establishing a bedtime routine, creating a calming sleep environment, and limiting screen time before bed.

Remember, a healthy lifestyle during the second trimester is about nourishing both your body and mind. Prioritize exercise, proper nutrition, and sufficient rest to ensure the best possible outcome for you and your baby. Embrace this special time as an opportunity to care for yourself and bond with your little one. With a healthy lifestyle, you'll be nurturing a strong foundation for the exciting journey of motherhood that lies ahead. Congratulations on taking proactive steps to care for yourself and your baby during this significant phase of your pregnancy!

Preparing for Parenting
(Building a Safe and Informed Foundation)

- **Parenting Classes and Workshops**
- **Babyproofing Your Home**

Welcome to the chapter dedicated to Preparing for Parenting! In this chapter, we will explore the importance of parenting classes and workshops to equip you with valuable knowledge and skills for parenthood. Additionally, we'll discuss the essential steps to babyproofing your home, ensuring a safe and nurturing environment for your little one.

Parenting Classes and Workshops

Parenting classes and workshops are wonderful resources that provide valuable insights and guidance for expectant parents. Let's explore the benefits of participating in these programs:

a) Knowledge and Information

Parenting classes offer a wealth of knowledge about newborn care, breastfeeding, infant safety, and other essential topics. They empower you with the information needed to make informed decisions for your baby.

b) Confidence Building

Attending parenting classes can boost your confidence as a new parent. You'll learn practical skills and gain reassurance that you are well-prepared for the arrival of your little one.

c) Connecting with Other Parents

These classes provide an opportunity to connect with other expectant parents. Sharing experiences and learning together can create a supportive community as you navigate parenthood.

d) Professional Guidance

Parenting classes are often led by experienced instructors, including healthcare providers and parenting experts, who can answer your questions and offer expert advice.

e) Bonding with Your Partner

Participating in parenting classes together allows you and your partner to strengthen your bond as you prepare for this new chapter in your lives.

Babyproofing Your Home

Creating a safe environment for your baby is of utmost importance. Babyproofing your home ensures that potential hazards are minimized. Here are some essential steps to consider:

a) Securing Furniture

Anchor heavy furniture, such as dressers and book-shelves, to the wall to prevent them from tipping over.

b) Electrical Outlets and Cords

Cover electrical outlets with safety plugs and use cord organizers to keep cords out of your baby's reach.

c) Stair Safety

Install safety gates at the top and bottom of staircases to prevent falls.

d) Cabinets and Drawers

Use childproof locks on cabinets and drawers to keep hazardous items, such as cleaning supplies, out of your baby's reach.

e) Window Safety

Install window guards or stops to prevent falls and keep blind cords out of reach.

f) Soft Surfaces

Place soft, cushioned mats on the floor to provide a safe play area for your baby.

g) Baby Monitor

Invest in a reliable baby monitor to keep an eye on your little one while they sleep or play in another room.

h) Safe Sleep Environment

Follow safe sleep guidelines by placing your baby on their back in a crib or bassinet with no loose bedding or soft toys.

By taking these precautionary measures, you can create a safe and nurturing environment for your baby to explore and grow.

Remember, preparing for parenting is an exciting and transformative process. Engaging in parenting classes and workshops equips you with knowledge and skills, fostering confidence and empowering you as a new parent. Babyproofing your home demonstrates your dedication to creating a safe haven for your little one. Embrace this journey with open arms, knowing that you are building a strong foundation for a loving and nurturing relationship with your child. Congratulations on taking proactive steps to prepare for the beautiful adventure of parenthood!

Chapter 5: The Third Trimester: Preparing for Birth

Coping with Physical Changes

- **Dealing with Weight Gain and Body Image**
- **Addressing Common Discomforts**

Welcome to the chapter dedicated to the Third Trimester of your pregnancy! In this chapter, we will explore the unique phase of preparing for birth while coping with the physical changes that come with it. We'll discuss ways to embrace your changing body and address common discomforts, ensuring a smooth transition as you approach the final stage of your pregnancy journey.

Dealing with Wight Gain and Body Image

As your baby grows and your body prepares for childbirth, weight gain is a natural part of the process. Here's how to navigate this phase with a positive outlook

a) Focus on Health and Nourishment

Remind yourself that weight gain during pregnancy is essential for your baby's growth and well-being. Focus on nourishing your body with a balanced diet and maintaining a healthy lifestyle.

b) Embrace the Beauty of Pregnancy

Recognize the beauty of the pregnancy journey and the miraculous work your body is doing to nurture new life. Embracing these changes can help you feel more confident and content.

c) Engage in Gentle Exercise

Staying active with gentle exercises like prenatal yoga or walking can support your physical and emotional well-being.

d) Seek Support from Loved Ones

Share your feelings with your partner, friends, or family members. Surrounding yourself with a supportive network can boost your self-esteem and ease any anxieties.

e) Wear Comfortable Clothing

Choose comfortable and flattering maternity wear that makes you feel good about yourself.

Addressing Common Discomforts

During the third trimester, some common discomforts may arise due to your body's adjustments. Here are strategies to manage them:

a) Back Pain

Use pillows for support while sitting or sleeping and practice good posture. Consider a maternity support belt to alleviate back strain.

b) Swollen Feet and Ankles

Elevate your legs when resting, avoid standing for long periods, and wear comfortable shoes.

c) Shortness of Breath

As your baby grows and takes up more space in your abdomen, you may experience shortness of breath. Practice deep breathing exercises to help manage this discomfort.

d) Difficulty Sleeping

Experiment with different sleep positions and use pillows for support. Establish a calming bedtime routine to promote better sleep.

e) Frequent Urination

Frequent bathroom trips are common in the third trimester. Stay hydrated, but try limiting fluid intake before bedtime to reduce nighttime awakenings.

f) Braxton Hicks Contractions

These are mild contractions that prepare your body for labor. Stay hydrated and change positions if they become uncomfortable. If you experience regular, strong contractions, contact your healthcare provider.

Remember, the third trimester is a period of preparation and anticipation for the birth of your baby. Embrace the changes happening in your body as you get closer to meeting your little ones. Focus on self-care and seek support from your healthcare provider and loved ones as needed. By addressing common discomforts and nurturing your body, you can create a positive and empowering experience in the final stages of your pregnancy. Congratulations on approaching the exciting milestone of bringing your baby into the world!

The Final Countdown
(Preparing for the Arrival of Your Baby)

- **Recognizing Signs of Labor**
- **Preparing for the Big Day - Packing Your Hospital Bag**

Welcome to the chapter dedicated to the Final Countdown of your pregnancy! In this chapter, we will explore the signs of labor that indicate your baby's imminent arrival and guide you through the essential steps of preparing for the big day by packing your hospital bag. As you approach the end of your pregnancy journey, it's crucial to be informed and ready for this momentous event.

Recognizing Signs of Labor

The final weeks of pregnancy are an exciting time as you await the arrival of your little one. Here are some signs that labor may be approaching:

a) Braxton Hicks Contractions

You may experience irregular, mild contractions, known as Braxton Hicks contractions, which are your body's way of preparing for labor.

b) Mucus Plug

The mucus plug, a thick discharge that seals the cervix during pregnancy, may be expelled as labor nears. This can happen a few days before labor begins.

c) Water Breaking

Your water may break, which is the release of amniotic fluid, signaling that labor is starting. This can happen as a sudden gush or a slow leak.

d) Cervical Changes

Your cervix may start to dilate and efface (thin out) as labor approaches. Your healthcare provider will check these changes during prenatal visits.

e) Nesting Instinct

Some women experience a burst of energy and an urge to tidy up and prepare for the baby's arrival, known as the nesting instinct.

Preparing for the Big Day - Packing Your Hospital Bag

Having a well-prepared hospital bag can bring peace of mind and ensure you have everything you need when it's time to go to the hospital. Here's a checklist of essential items to pack.

a) Personal Identification and Medical Documents

Bring your ID, health insurance card, and any necessary medical documents, such as your prenatal records.

b) Comfortable Clothing

Pack comfortable, loose-fitting clothes to wear during labor and after delivery.

c) Toiletries

Include toiletries like a toothbrush, toothpaste, shampoo, conditioner, and any other personal care items.

d) Snacks and Drinks

Bring some light snacks and drinks to keep you energized during labor.

e) Entertainment and Relaxation

Consider bringing items like books, magazines, music, or other forms of entertainment to help pass the time and relax.

f) Nursing Supplies

If you plan to breastfeed, bring nursing bras, nursing pads, and lanolin cream.

g) Baby Essentials

Pack clothing for the baby, receiving blankets, diapers, wipes, and a going-home outfit.

h) Car Seat

Make sure you have a properly installed car seat to safely transport your baby home.

Remember, every pregnancy and labor experience is unique. While it's essential to be prepared, try to stay flexible and open to the unpredictability of childbirth. Trust your body and the support of your healthcare provider and birthing team. By recognizing the signs of labor and having your hospital bag ready, you can approach the final countdown with confidence and excitement. Congratulations on reaching this momentous stage of your pregnancy journey and preparing to welcome your precious bundle of joy into the world!

Birth Plans and Delivery Options
(Empowering Your Birth Experience)

- **Understanding Birth Plans**
- **Considering Natural vs. Medical Interventions**

Welcome to the chapter dedicated to Birth Plans and Delivery Options! In this chapter, we will explore the significance of birth plans and how they can help you have a positive and empowering birth experience. Additionally, we'll discuss the differences between natural and medical interventions during childbirth, enabling you to make informed decisions that align with your preferences and needs.

Understanding Birth Plans

A birth plan is a written document that outlines your preferences and wishes for the labor and delivery process. Creating a birth plan can be a valuable tool for communicating your desires to your healthcare provider and birthing team. Here's how to develop an effective birth plan:

a) Communicate with Your Healthcare Provider

Start by having open and honest conversations with your healthcare provider about your preferences for childbirth. They can provide valuable guidance and address any concerns you may have.

b) *Include Your Birth Preferences*

Your birth plan should reflect your preferences for pain management, birthing positions, who you want present during labor, and any other aspects of the birth experience that are important to you.

c) *Be Flexible*

While a birth plan can help guide your decisions, remember that labor and delivery can be unpredictable. Be open to adjustments and changes as needed.

d) *Discuss Your Birth Plan with Your Birthing Team*

Share your birth plan with your birthing team well in advance of your due date. This way, they can review and understand your preferences, ensuring a cohesive approach to your care.

Considering Natural vs. Medical Interventions

As you prepare for childbirth, you may hear about different approaches to managing labor and delivery. It's essential to understand the differences between natural and medical interventions:

a) *Natural Interventions*

Natural childbirth involves minimal medical interventions and aims to let labor progress without interference. Techniques like relaxation, breathing exercises, movement, and positioning can help manage pain.

b) Medical Interventions

Medical interventions, such as pain medication, epidurals, and assisted deliveries (forceps or vacuum extraction), are available to manage pain and assist with the birthing process. These interventions can be valuable in specific situations but may not align with everyone's birth preferences.

c) Informed Decision Making

The key to making informed decisions is understanding both natural and medical interventions, along with their potential benefits and risks. Your healthcare provider can help you weigh these options based on your individual circumstances.

d) Flexibility and Open Communication

It's crucial to approach your birth plan with flexibility and to keep an open line of communication with your healthcare provider. Be prepared to adapt your plan based on how labor progresses and any unforeseen circumstances that may arise.

Remember, your birth experience is personal and unique to you. By creating a birth plan that reflects your preferences and understanding your options for natural and medical interventions, you can empower yourself to make informed decisions during childbirth. Trust in your body's ability to bring your baby into the world, and rely on the support and expertise of your birthing team. Embrace this transformative moment with confidence, knowing that you are an active participant in the birth of your child. Congratulations on taking proactive steps to shape a birth experience that honors your choices and priorities!

Preparing Emotionally for Labor and Delivery
(Nurturing a Positive Mindset)

- **Addressing Fears and Anxieties**
- **Creating a Calm and Positive Birth Environment**

Welcome to the chapter dedicated to Preparing Emotionally for Labor and Delivery! In this chapter, we will explore the essential steps to address fears and anxieties surrounding childbirth and create a calm and positive birth environment. By nurturing a positive mindset, you can approach labor and delivery with confidence and inner strength.

Addressing Fears and Anxieties

As the due date approaches, it's common to experience a mix of emotions, including fears and anxieties about labor and delivery. Here's how to address these feelings:

a) Seek Information and Knowledge

Educate yourself about the labor and delivery process. Attend childbirth classes, read books, and talk to other mothers about their experiences. Being well-informed can alleviate uncertainties and empower you.

b) Communicate with Your Healthcare Provider

Discuss your fears and concerns with your healthcare provider openly. They can provide reassurance, address your questions, and offer guidance to ease your worries.

c) Practice Relaxation Techniques

Learn relaxation techniques such as deep breathing, visualization, and mindfulness. These practices can help you stay calm and centered during labor.

d) Consider a Birth Plan

Creating a birth plan that reflects your preferences and desires can give you a sense of control and direction during the birthing process.

e) Talk to Your Support System

Share your feelings with your partner, family, or friends. Having a support system that understands and listens can be incredibly comforting.

Creating a Calm and Positive Birth Environment

The birthing environment plays a significant role in how you experience labor and delivery. Here's how to create a calm and positive space for this transformative event:

a) Choose a Supportive Birth Location

Consider giving birth in a setting where you feel comfortable and supported, whether it's a hospital, birthing center, or home birth with a midwife.

b) Bring Comfort Items

Pack comforting items in your hospital bag, such as a favorite blanket, pillow, or soothing music.

c) Dim Lighting and Relaxing Music

Creating a calming atmosphere with dim lighting and soft, relaxing music can help you feel more at ease during labor.

d) Encourage Positive Affirmations

Write down positive affirmations that resonate with you and read them aloud during labor. These affirmations can instill confidence and positivity.

e) Utilize Aromatherapy

Some women find aromatherapy helpful during labor. Consider bringing essential oils that promote relaxation and tranquility.

f) Involve Your Birth Partner

Your birth partner can play a crucial role in creating a positive birth environment. Discuss with them how they can support and encourage you during labor.

Remember, emotional preparation for labor and delivery is just as important as physical preparation. Acknowledge and address your fears, and take proactive steps to nurture a calm and positive mindset. Surround yourself with a supportive birthing team and environment that aligns with your preferences. Trust in the strength of your body and the love and support of your loved ones. As you embrace the upcoming journey of childbirth, know that you are capable and resilient, and you have everything within you to experience a positive and empowering birth.

Chapter 6: Labor and Delivery
Stages of Labor
(Navigating the Path to Birth)

- **Early Labor: Signs and Coping Strategies**
- **Active Labor: The Main Event**
- **Transition and Pushing**

Welcome to the chapter dedicated to the Stags of Labor! In this chapter, we will explore the different stages of labor and the experiences you can expect during each phase. By understanding these stages and employing effective coping strategies, you can approach labor with confidence and inner strength.

Early Labor: Signs and Coping Strategies

a) Signs of Early Labor

Early labor is the initial phase of the birthing process. It is characterized by mild contractions that may feel like menstrual cramps, lower back discomfort, or a sensation of pressure. You may also notice the loss of your mucus plug or a slight trickle of amniotic fluid.

b) Coping Strategies for Early Labor

During early labor, focus on relaxation and staying hydrated. Practice deep breathing, take warm baths, or use relaxation techniques to manage any discomfort. Engage in light activities to distract yourself and conserve energy for the active phase of labor.

Active Labor: The Main Event

a) Signs of Active Labor

Active labor marks the beginning of more intense and frequent contractions. Your cervix will continue to dilate, and the pace of labor will pick up. Contractions may become longer, stronger, and closer together, usually lasting 60-90 seconds and occurring every 3-5 minutes.

b) Coping Strategies for Active Labor

During active labor, focus on staying focused and calm. Use relaxation techniques, such as controlled breathing and visualization, to manage the intensity of contractions. Find comfort in changing positions, walking, or using a birthing ball to help your baby move down the birth canal.

Transition and Pushing

a) Transition Phase

Transition is the final phase of labor before pushing begins. During this stage, contractions may be extremely intense and close together. You may experience feelings of doubt, fatigue, and heightened emotions.

b) Coping Strategies for Transition

Transition can be challenging, but remember that it is a sign that you are getting closer to meeting your baby. Stay focused and motivated by reminding yourself of the progress you have made. Lean on your support system for encouragement and reassurance.

c) Pushing Phase

The pushing phase begins when your cervix is fully dilated, and you feel the urge to push. This stage requires focused effort and determination as you work with your body to guide your baby through the birth canal.

d) Coping Strategies for Pushing

Listen to your body and work with your healthcare provider's guidance. Push when you feel the urge and rest between contractions. Focus on your baby's arrival, knowing that each push brings you closer to meeting them.

Remember, every labor experience is unique. Trust in the strength of your body and the support of your birthing team. Employ coping strategies that work best for you, and don't hesitate to communicate your needs and preferences throughout the process. By understanding the stages of labor and using effective coping strategies, you can navigate the path to birth with courage and determination. Congratulations on preparing for this extraordinary journey of bringing new life into the world!

Delivery Methods
(Understanding Birth Options)

- **Vaginal Birth vs. Cesarean Section**
- **Assisted Deliveries: Forceps and Vacuum Extraction**

Welcome to the chapter dedicated to Delivery Methods! In this chapter, we will explore the different options for giving birth and the circumstances in which each method may be used. Understanding delivery methods can help you make informed decisions that align with your preferences and ensure the safe arrival of your baby.

Vaginal Birth vs. Cesarean Section

a) Vaginal Birth

Vaginal birth is the most common and natural method of childbirth. During a vaginal birth, your baby is born through the birth canal. This process can be aided by your body's natural contractions and pushing efforts.

Advantages of Vaginal Birth

- Generally, a shorter recovery time compared to a cesarean section.
- There is a lower risk of certain complications associated with major surgery.

b) Cesarean Section (C-section)

A cesarean section is a surgical procedure in which your baby is delivered through an incision made in your abdomen and uterus. C-sections are typically recommended for specific medical reasons, such as certain pregnancy complications or when vaginal birth is not safe for you or your baby.

Advantages of Cesarean Section

- Planned cesarean sections can be scheduled, offering predictability for the birth.
- It may be necessary for certain medical conditions to ensure the well-being of you and your baby.

Assisted Deliveries: Forceps and Vacuum Extraction

a) Forceps Delivery

A forceps delivery is an assisted vaginal birth method in which curved, tong-like instruments are used to gently guide your baby's head through the birth canal. Forceps may be used if there are concerns about your baby's well-being during labor or if you are having difficulty pushing.

b) Vacuum Extraction

Vacuum extraction is another assisted vaginal birth method. A soft cup is placed on your baby's head, and suction is used to help guide your baby through the birth canal during contractions. Vacuum extraction is typically considered if there is a need for a prompt delivery or if you are experiencing exhaustion during the pushing phase.

It's important to note that the decision regarding the deliv-ery method is made based on various factors, including your medical history, the well-being of you and your baby, and the progress of labor.

Remember, each birthing experience is unique, and there is no ones-size-fits-all approach to childbirth. Your healthcare provider will work with you to determine the most appropriate delivery method based on your individual circumstances. Being well-informed about the different options can help you feel more prepared and empowered as you approach the delivery of your baby. Embrace the upcoming birth with confidence, knowing that you are in capable hands and that the priority is the safe and healthy arrival of your precious little one. Congratulations on taking proactive steps to understand your birthing options and prepare for this extraordinary moment of bringing new life into the world!

Pain Management Techniques

- **Medication Options**
- **Natural Pain Relief Methods**

Welcome to the chapter dedicated to Pain Management Techniques during labor and delivery! In this chapter, we will explore different methods to manage pain during childbirth, including medication options and natural pain relief methods. By understanding these techniques, you can make informed choices that support your comfort and well-being throughout the birthing process.

Medication Options

a) Epidural Analgesia

An epidural is a common pain relief option during labor. It involves the insertion of a small catheter into your lower back, allowing a continuous flow of pain-reliving medication near the nerves that transmit labor pain. Epidurals can provide significant pain relief while allowing you to remain awake and actively participate in the birthing process.

Advantages of Epidural Analgesia

- Provides effective pain relief during labor.
- Allows you to conserve energy for the pushing phase.

b) IV Pain Medications

Intravenous (IV) pain medications,   such as opioids, can be administered to help manage pain during labor. These medications can provide temporary relief and may be useful for women who prefer not to have an epidural or for those in the early stages of labor.

Advantages of IV Pain Medications

- Quick pain relief during labor.
- Can be useful for managing pain before an epidural is administered.

Natural Pain Relief Methods

a) Movement and Positioning

Changing positions, walking, rocking, or swaying can help ease discomfort during labor. Finding a position that feels comfortable can aid the progress of labor and reduce pres-sure on certain areas of your body.

b) Breathing Techniques

Practicing controlled breathing can promote relaxation and help manage pain during contractions. Deep breathing, rhythmic breathing, or guided breathing techniques can be beneficial.

c) Water Therapy

Using a birthing pool or taking a warm shower can offer soothing relief during labor. Water therapy can help you relax and cop with contractions.

d) Massage and Counter Pressure

Gentle massage from your birth partner or a trained doula can provide comfort and relaxation during labor. Applying pressure to specific areas, such as your lower back or hips, can help alleviate pain.

e) Relaxation Techniques

Mindfulness, visualization, or guided imagery can help you focus and stay calm during labor. These techniques can re-duce anxiety and crate a more positive birthing experience.

Remember, pain management during labor is a personal choice, and there is no right or wrong way to approach it. Each woman's pain tolerance and preferences are unique. Discuss your options with your healthcare provider and cre-ate a birth plan that aligns with your needs and desires. Keep an open mind, as labor can by unpredictable, and you may decide to try different pain relief methods throughout the process. Embrace the support of your birthing team and your loved ones, knowing that they are there to encourage and empower you every step of the way. Congratulations on preparing for a positive and empower-ing birth experience, where your comfort

and well-being are at the forefront of this transformative moment!

The Miracle of Birth
(Embracing the Arrival of Your Baby)

- **Meeting Your Baby for the First Time**
- **The Golden Hour: Bonding and Breast-feeding**

Welcome to the chapter dedicated to The Miracle of Birth! In this chapter, we will explore the precious moments of meeting your baby for the first time and the significance of the Golden Hour, a special time for bonding and breast-feeding. These moments are filled with wonder, love, and the beginning of a beautiful journey with your newborn.

Meeting Your Baby for the First Time

a) The Moment of Birth

As labor finishes, the moment of birth arrives. Your hard work and resilience throughout the birthing process lead to the joyous moment when your baby arrive into the world.

b) Emotions Overflow

Meeting your baby for the first time is an overwhelming and motional experience. You may feel a surge of love, joy, and a deep sense of connection with your newborn.

c) Skin-to-Skin Contact

After birth, placing your baby on your chest for skin-to-skin contact is a heartwarming way to welcome them into the world. This physical closeness helps regulate your baby's body temperature, heart rate, and breathing while strength-ening the bond between you both.

d) Discovering Your Baby

Take the time to observe and marvel at your baby's features, tiny hands, and feet. These early moments crate a lasting impression of your baby's unique char-acteristics.

The Golden Hour: Bonding and Breastfeeding

a) The Golden Hour

The first hour after birth is often referred to as the Golden hour, as it is a critical time for bonding and establishing breastfeeding.

b) Bonding with Your Baby

During the Golden Hour, focus on nurturing your bond with your baby through skin-to-skin contact, eye contact, and gentle touch. Your baby is comforted by the familiar sound of your voice and the rhythm of your heartbeat.

c) Initiating Breastfeeding

The Golden Hour is an opportune time to initiate breast-feeding if you choose to breastfeed. Your baby is often alert and ready to feed during this time. Skin-to-skin con-tact can encourage your baby to latch on and begin breast-feeding successfully.

d) *Support from Your Birthing Team*

Your healthcare provider and birthing team can assist you in making the most of the Golden Hour. They can offer guidance on breastfeeding positions, help with latching, and provide support as you begin your breastfeeding journey.

e) *Respect Your Preferences*

While the Golden Hour is beneficial, it's essential to respect your preferences and needs. If you need additional rest or medical attention, you can still bond with your baby and initiate breastfeeding at a later time.

Remember, the Miracle of Birth marks the beginning of an incredible journey of motherhood. Cherish the early moments of meeting your baby, as they are precious and fleet-ing. Embrace the Golden Hour as a time of connection and bonding, setting the foundation for a strong and loving re-lationship with your newborn. Trust in your instincts and the support of your healthcare provider and birthing team as you navigate these early moments of parenthood. Congratulations on welcoming your baby into the world, and may this extraordinary journey of motherhood be filled with love, joy, and treasured memories!

Chapter 7: The Fourth Trimester: Postpartum Care and Beyond

The Postpartum Period

- **Physical Recovery and Healing**
- **Emotional Well-being: Baby Blues vs. Postpartum Depression**

Welcome to the chapter dedicated to The Postpartum Peri-od! In this chapter, we will explore the importance of physical recovery and haling after childbirth and discuss emotional well-being, including the differences between baby blues and postpartum depression. This period is a time of adjustment and self-care as you embark on the journey of motherhood.

Physical Recovery and Healing

a) Rest and Self-Care

During the postpartum period, prioritize rest and self-care. Your body has undergone significant changes during pregnancy and childbirth, and it needs time to heal.

b) Managing Postpartum Discomforts

You may experience discomforts such as vaginal soreness, perineal tears, or cesarean section incision haling. Follow your healthcare provider's guidance on pain management and caring for these areas.

c) Pelvic Floor Exercises

Pelvic floor exercises, often referred to as Kegel exercises, can help strengthen your pelvic muscles and promote heal-ing.

d) Nutrition and Hydration

Maintain a balanced diet and stay hydrated to support your body's recovery and breastfeeding journey.

e) Reach Out for Support

Don't hesitate to seek support from your partner, family, or friends during this time. They can assist with household tasks and caring for the baby, allowing you to focus on healing.

Emotional Well-being: Baby Blues vs. Postpartum Depression

a) Baby Blues

The baby blues are common and usually occur within the first two weeks after childbirth. You may experience mood swings, irritability, and tearfulness. These feelings are often transient and can be attributed to hormonal changes, exhaustion, and adjusting to the demands of motherhood.

b) Coping with Baby Blues

To cope with baby blues, prioritize rest, talk to your partner or loved ones about your feelings, and allow yourself to express motions without judgment.

c) Postpartum Depression (PPD)

Postpartum depression is a more prolonged and severe con-dition that affects some new mothers. PPD may include persistent feelings of sadness, loss of interest in activities, changes in appetite, sleep disturbances, and difficulty bonding with the baby.

d) Seeking Help for Postpartum Depression

If you suspect you may be experiencing postpartum depres-sion, don't hesitate to seek professional help. Your healthcare provider can offer guidance and support, and they may recommend counseling, therapy, or medication if needed.

e) Supportive Environment

Creating a supportive environment and seeking help when needed can significantly improve your motional well-being during the postpartum period.

Remember, the postpartum period is a time of adjustment and recovery. Be gentle with yourself as you navigate the physical and emotional changes that come with mother-hood. Prioritize self-care, rest, and seeking support when needed. Reach out to your healthcare provider or a mental health professional if you have concerns about your motional well-being. Embrace this transformative period with love and patience, knowing that it is a time of growth and bonding with your baby. Congratulations on becoming a mother and embarking on this beautiful journey of nurturing and caring for your little one!

Newborn Care and Parenting Tips
(Nurturing Your Little One and Yourself)

- **Nurturing Your Baby's Development**
- **Sleep Routines and Self-Care for Parents**

Welcome to the chapter dedicated to Newborn Care and Parenting Tips! In this chapter, we will explore essential ways to nurture your baby's development and create sleep routines, as well as the importance of self-care for parents. These tips will guide you through the early days of parenthood, helping you build a strong bond with your newborn while taking care of yourself.

Nurturing Your Baby's Development

a) Bonding and Skin-to-Skin Contact

Continue to nurture your bond with your baby through fre-quent skin-to-skin contact and cuddling. Physical closeness helps your baby feel secure and loved.

b) Feeding and Nutrition

Whether you choose to breastfeed or use formula, en-sure your baby is getting the nourishment they need. Follow your healthcare provider's guidance on feeding and track your baby's growth and weight gain.

c) Responding to Your Baby's Cues

Learn to recognize your baby's cues for hunger, sleep, and comfort. Responding promptly to their needs fosters a sense of security and trust.

d) Tummy Time and Motor Skills

Engage your baby in supervised tummy time to help them strengthen their neck and upper body muscles. Encourage reaching and grasping as your baby starts to explore their environment.

e) Encourage Sensory Stimulation

Expose your baby to different textures, sounds, and sights to encourage their sensory development. Soft toys, rattles, and gentle music can be enjoyable for your little one.

Sleep Routines and Self-Care for Parents

a) Establish a Sleep Routine

Creating a consistent bedtime routine can help your baby recognize when it's time to sleep. A warm bath, gentle mas-sage, or reading a bedtime story can signal that it's time for rest.

b) Napping Patterns

Newborns sleep a lot, but their sleep patterns can be irregu-lar. Allow your baby to nap when they are tired, and follow their lead for nap times during the day.

c) Taking Care of Yourself

Parenting can be demanding, so it's essential to take care of yourself. Prioritize self-care by resting when your baby sleeps, eating nourishing meals, and seeking support from family or friends.

d) Ask for Help

Don't hesitate to ask for help if you need it. Whether it's assistance with baby care or someone to talk to, reaching out to your support system can make a significant differ-ence.

e) Accepting Imperfections

Parenting is a learning process, and its okay to make mis-takes or face challenges. Be kind to yourself and remember that nobody is a perfect parent.

Remember, every baby is unique, and there is no one-size-fits-all approach to parenting. Listen to your instincts, trust your judgment, and be patient with yourself and your baby. Cherish the precious moments of bonding and discovery with your new-born. As you care for your little one, don't forget to care for yourself as well. Prioritize self-care, seek support when needed, and embrace the joys and chal-lenges of parenthood with love and grace. Congratulations on be-coming a parent and embarking on this incredible journey of nurturing and guiding your precious baby!

Breastfeeding and Bottle-Feeding
(Nourishing Your Baby with Love)

- **Latching and Nursing Techniques**
- **Choosing and Using Baby Formula**

Welcome to the chapter dedicated to Breastfeeding and Bottle-Feeding! In this chapter, we will explore the im-portance of latching and nursing techniques for breastfeeding, as well as the considerations for choosing and using baby formula for bottle-feeding. These feeding methods provide your baby with the nourishment they need to grow and thrive, while also fostering a strong bond between you and your little one.

Breastfeeding

a) Latching and Nursing Techniques

Proper latching is essential for successful breastfeeding. Here are some tips for latching and nursing your baby

- ***Find a comfortable position***: Sit or lie in a position that supports your back and arms while keeping your baby close to your breast.
- ***Aim for a wide latch***: Encourage your baby to open their mouth wide and take in as much of the areola (the dark area around the nipple) as possible.

- ***Listen for swallowing***: As your baby nurses, listen for soft, rhythmic swallowing sounds, which indi-cate they are effectively feeding.
- ***Establish an feeding schedule***: In the early days, breastfeed your baby on demand, which may be every 2-3 hours. As your baby grows, they will es-tablish their own feeding routine.

b) Benefits of Breastfeeding

Breast milk is tailored to meet your baby's specific needs, providing essential nutrients and antibodies that support their immune system. Breastfeeding also enhances the bond between you and your baby and has various health benefits for both of you.

c) Overcoming Challenges

Breastfeeding can sometimes come with challenges, such as sore nipples or difficulty latching. Seek guid-ance and sup-port from a lactation consultant or a healthcare provider if you encounter any difficulties.

Bottle-Feeding

a) Choosing Baby Formula

If you choose to bottle-feed, selecting the right baby for-mula is important. Speak with your healthcare provider about the best formula option for your baby. Most baby formulas are made with cow's milk, soy, or other ingredi-ents suitable for infants.

b) Preparing Baby Formula

Follow the instructions on the formula packaging to ensure you prepare the formula correctly.

Use clean, sterilized bottles and nipples for feeding.

c) Feeding Time

Hold your baby close while feeding and make eye contact to encourage bonding. Allow your baby to feed at their own pace, pausing and burping as needed.

d) Sterilizing Equipment

For the first few months, it's essential to sterilize bottles, nipples, and other feeding equipment to maintain hygiene and prevent infections.

e) Bonding During Bottle-Feeding

Although bottle-feeding is different from breastfeeding, it still provides an opportunity for bonding. Cuddle your baby and talk to them while they feed to strengthen your connec-tion.

Remember, both breastfeeding and bottle-feeding can be nurturing experiences for you and your baby. The choice between the two methods is personal and should align with your preferences and circum-stances. Whatever method you choose, approach feeding time with love, patience, and at-tentiveness. Seek support and guidance if needed, and cherish the precious moments of nourishing and caring for your little one. Congratulations on providing your baby with the love and nourishment they need to grow into a healthy and happy child!

Balancing Work and Motherhood
(Nurturing Your Career and Family)

- **Returning to Work: Challenges and Solutions**
- **Maintaining a Healthy Work-Life Balance**

Welcome to the chapter dedicated to Balancing Work and Motherhood! In this chapter, we will explore the challenges and solutions for returning to work after having a baby and maintaining a healthy work-life balance as a new mother. Balancing these important aspects of your life can be both rewarding and demanding, but with thoughtful planning and support, you can create a fulfilling and harmonious rou-tine.

Returning to Work: Challenges and Solutions

a) Emotional Challenges

Returning to work after maternity leave can be emo-tionally challenging. You may experience feelings of guilt, worry, or separation anxiety. Know that it is entirely normal to have these emotions as you adjust to being away from your baby.

Solution: Seek Support and Communication

Talk to your employer about your concerns and explore flexible work options, such as part-time or telecommuting. Establish open communication with your colleagues and supervisors, so they understand your needs as a new moth-er.

b) Childcare Arrangements

Finding suitable childcare can be a major concern for work-ing mothers. Research different childcare options, such as daycare centers or hiring a nanny, and choose what aligns best with your family's needs and values.

Solution: Plan Ahead

Start looking for childcare early, and visit potential provid-ers to ensure they meet your criteria. Having a reliable and trusted childcare arrangement will ease your mind while you're at work.

Maintaining a Healthy Work-Life Balance

a) Time Management

Balancing work and motherhood requires effective time management. Prioritize tasks both at work and at home, and be realistic about what you can accomplish in a day.

Solution: Create a Schedule

Establish a daily or weekly schedule that includes dedicat-ed time for work, family, and self-care. Organizing your time can help you feel more in control and reduce stress.

b) Boundaries

Setting boundaries is essential for maintaining a healthy work-life balance. Avoid overcommitting at work and be mindful of taking on additional responsibilities that may interfere with your family time.

Solution: Learn to Say No

Don't be afraid to say no when your plate is already full. Communicate your limits to your employer and colleagues to ensure they respect your work-life balance.

c) Self-Care

As a working mother, it's crucial to take care of your own well-being. Make time for activities that rejuvenate you, such as exercise, hobbies, or spending quality time with your partner.

Solution: Delegate and Accept Help

Delegate household tasks and accept help from your part-ner, family, or friends. Remember that it's okay to ask for assistance when needed.

Remember, balancing work and motherhood is an ongoing journey of adjustments and learning. Each day may present new challenges and opportunities for growth. Trust your-self, seek support from loved ones, and be kind to yourself as you navigate this path.

You are a strong and capable mother, and with a balanced approach to work and family life, you can flourish both personally and professionally. Congratulations on embarking on this remarkable journey of juggling the joys of motherhood and your career!

Conclusion- Embracing Your Journey into Motherhood

(Reflections on the Journey)

- **Celebrating Your Transformation into Motherhood**
- **Embracing the Future: Parenting with Confidence**

Congratulations on completing this essential guide to first-time pregnancy and motherhood! Throughout this book, we have explored the miraculous journey of pregnancy, the joys and challenges of childbirth, and the nurturing care of your newborn. As we conclude this chapter, let's reflect on the transformation into motherhood and the exciting future ahead as you embrace parenting with confidence.

Celebrating Your Transformation into Motherhood

a) A Journey of Growth

From the moment you learned you were expecting to the miracle of birth, you have embarked on a journey of growth and transformation. Each step of this journey has shaped you into the strong and nurturing mother you are today.

b) Embracing Motherhood

Motherhood is a profound experience that opens your heart to a love like no other. It is a journey of discovery, learning, and adapting to the ever-changing needs of your baby.

c) Cherishing Moments

Take the time to cherish the precious moments with your baby – the gentle touch of their tiny hand, the first smile, and the warmth of their presence. These moments are short lived, and they form the foundation of your deep bond with your little one.

Embracing the Future: Parenting with Confidence

a) Trusting Your Instincts

As a parent, you will face many decisions and challenges along the way. Trust your instincts and intuition, for you know what is best for your child.

b) Learning and Growing Together

Parenting is a continuous journey of learning and growing, both for you and your child. Embrace the joy of discovery as you navigate each phase of your baby's development.

c) Creating a Supportive Network

Build a supportive network of family, friends, and other parents. Sharing experiences and seeking advice can be in-valuable as you navigate the joys and challenges of parenthood.

d) Self-Care

Remember the importance of self-care. Taking care of your-self enables you to be the best version of yourself for your baby.

e) Celebrating Milestones

Celebrate every milestone, big and small, in your baby's life. Each achievement is a witness to their growth and the love and care you provide.

In conclusion, the journey of first-time pregnancy and motherhood is a momentous and transformative experience. As you navigate this path, remember that it's okay to seek help, to ask questions, and to learn along the way. Trust in your abilities as a mother, for your love and care are the most precious gifts you can give to your child. Embrace the adventure of parenting with confidence, knowing that you are shaping a bright future for your little one. Congratulations on becoming a mother, and may this beautiful journey be filled with joy, love, and cherished memories that will last a lifetime!

Appendix

Glossary of Pregnancy-related Terms

Below is a glossary of pregnancy-related terms with brief explanations in simple language for the book "Blossoming Maternity: Your Essential Guide to a First-Time Pregnancy":

Amniocentesis: A prenatal test where a small sample of amniotic fluid is taken to check for genetic disorders or other potential issues with the baby.

Amniotic Fluid: The fluid surrounding the baby inside the amniotic sac. It protects and cushions the baby during pregnancy.

Antenatal Care: Medical care and check-ups provided to pregnant women to monitor the health of both the mother and the baby.

Baby Bump: The visible roundness or protrusion of a pregnant woman's belly as the baby grows.

Breech Position: When the baby's buttocks or feet are positioned to come out first during birth instead of the head.

Braxton Hicks Contractions: Painless, irregular contractions felt during pregnancy that prepare the uterus for childbirth.

Cervix: The lower part of the uterus that opens during labor to allow the baby to pass through the birth canal.

Chorionic Villus Sampling (CVS): A prenatal test where a small tissue sample is taken from the placenta to check for genetic disorders in the baby.

Colostrum: The first milk produced by the breasts during pregnancy and after childbirth, rich in nutrients and antibodies for the baby.

Conception: The fertilization of an egg by sperm, leading to the beginning of pregnancy.

Contractions: The tightening and relaxing of the uterus during labor to help the baby move through the birth canal.

Crowning: The stage during childbirth when the baby's head becomes visible at the opening of the vagina.

Cesarean Section (C-Section): A surgical procedure to de-liver the baby through an incision in the abdomen and uter-us.

Cord Blood Banking: Collecting and storing umbilical cord blood for potential future medical use.

Cloth Diapers: Reusable diapers made from fabric, an eco-friendly alternative to disposable diapers.

Colic: A condition where a baby cries for extended periods, often due to digestive discomfort.

Compression Stockings: Specialized socks or stockings that help improve blood circulation and reduce swelling during pregnancy.

Contraction Timer: A tool or app used to track the frequency and duration of contractions during labor.

Doula: A trained professional who provides emotional and physical support to a woman during pregnancy, childbirth, and postpartum.

Due Date: The estimated date when the baby is expected to be born based on the first day of the last menstrual period.

Dilation: The opening of the cervix during labor to allow the baby to pass through the birth canal.

Ectopic Pregnancy: A pregnancy where the fertilized egg implants outside the uterus, usually in the fallopian tube.

Embryo: The early stage of development of the baby, from conception until about eight weeks of pregnancy.

Epidural: A form of pain relief used during labor, where medication is injected into the space around the spinal cord.

Effacement: The thinning and shortening of the cervix as it prepares for childbirth.

Engorgement: Swelling and discomfort of the breasts due to increased milk supply after childbirth.

Episiotomy: A surgical cut made during childbirth to widen the vaginal opening.

Fertility Awareness: Tracking menstrual cycles and body signs to identify fertile days for pregnancy planning.

Fetal Doppler: A handheld device used to listen to the baby's heartbeat during pregnancy.

Folic Acid: A B-vitamin important for preventing birth defects in the baby's brain and spine.

Fontanelles: Soft spots on the baby's head where the skull bones have not yet fused.

Fundal Height Measurement: The measurement of the height of the uterus to assess fetal growth during pregnancy.

Infant Care: The care and handling of a newborn baby, including feeding, diapering, and soothing techniques.

Fallopian Tubes: Tubes that carry the egg from the ovaries to the uterus. Fertilization occurs in the fallopian tubes.

Fetal Movement: The movements felt by the mother as the baby kicks, rolls, or stretches inside the womb.

Fetus: The developing baby from the ninth week of pregnancy until birth.

Full-Term: When a pregnancy reaches its normal duration, usually around 39 to 40 weeks.

Gestational Age: The age of the baby calculated from the first day of the last menstrual period.

Gestational Diabetes: A type of diabetes that develops during pregnancy and can affect the baby's health.

Gestational Hypertension: High blood pressure that develops during pregnancy and can be harmful if left untreated.

Glucose Tolerance Test (GTT): A test to check how well the body processes sugar and to detect gestational diabetes.

Group B Streptococcus (GBS) Screening: A test to check for the presence of a type of bacteria that can be harmful to the baby during childbirth.

HCG (Human Chorionic Gonadotropin): A hormone produced during pregnancy, which is detected in pregnancy tests.

Heartbeat: The rhythmic pumping of the baby's heart, usually heard during prenatal check-ups.

High-Risk Pregnancy: A pregnancy that has a higher chance of complications due to various factors such as health conditions or previous pregnancy issues.

Hormones: Chemical messengers produced during pregnancy that regulate various bodily functions and support the baby's growth.

Intrauterine Device (IUD): A birth control method that is placed in the uterus to prevent pregnancy.

Jaundice: A condition where the baby's skin and eyes may appear yellow due to excess bilirubin in the blood.

Kick Counts: Tracking and counting the baby's movements as a way to monitor their well-being during pregnancy.

Lamaze Technique: A method of childbirth education that focuses on relaxation and breathing techniques to manage labor pain.

Latch: The way a baby attaches to the mother's breast during breastfeeding.

Lightening: The sensation of the baby moving lower into the pelvis as labor approaches.

Lochia: Vaginal discharge after childbirth, which consists of blood, mucus, and uterine tissue.

Low Birth Weight: When a baby is born weighing less than 5.5 pounds, often requiring special care and monitoring.

Maternity Leave: Time off work given to expectant mothers before and after childbirth.

Meconium: The baby's first bowel movement, which is thick and dark green.

Miscarriage: The loss of a pregnancy before the 20th week, also known as a spontaneous abortion.

Morning Sickness: Nausea and vomiting commonly experienced during early pregnancy.

Multifetal Pregnancy: A pregnancy with more than one baby, such as twins, triplets, or higher-order multiples.

Nausea and Vomiting: Commonly experienced in the early stages of pregnancy, often referred to as morning sickness.

Neonate: A newborn baby in the first four weeks of life.

Nuchal Translucency (NT) Test: A prenatal screening test to assess the risk of chromosomal abnormalities, particularly Down syndrome.

Obstetrician: A doctor specializing in pregnancy, childbirth, and postpartum care.

Ovulation: The release of a mature egg from the ovary, typically occurring midway through the menstrual cycle.

Placenta: An organ that develops during pregnancy and provides nutrients and oxygen to the baby while removing waste products.

Postpartum Depression (PPD): A form of depression that some women experience after childbirth, characterized by feelings of sadness and anxiety.

Postpartum Period: The period after childbirth when the body undergoes physical and emotional changes.

Preconception Care: Medical care and lifestyle adjustments taken before pregnancy to ensure optimal health for the mother and baby.

Preeclampsia: A condition characterized by high blood pressure and damage to organs, usually occurring after 20 weeks of pregnancy.

Premature Birth: When a baby is born before 37 weeks of pregnancy, requiring special medical care.

Quickening: The first movements of the baby felt by the mother, usually occurring between 16 to 25 weeks of pregnancy.

Rh factor: A protein present on the surface of red blood cells that can cause complications if the mother's blood type is Rh-negative and the baby's blood type is Rh-positive.

Round Ligament Pain: A sharp or stabbing pain in the lower abdomen caused by the stretching of the round ligaments supporting the uterus.

Stillbirth: The loss of a baby after 20 weeks of pregnancy before birth.

Striae Gravidarum (Stretch Marks): Pink or purple lines that appear on the skin due to stretching during pregnancy.

Teratogens: Substances or agents that can cause birth defects or harm the developing baby during pregnancy.

Thrombosis: The formation of blood clots, which can be a concern during pregnancy due to hormonal changes.

Trimester: The three distinct periods of pregnancy, each lasting about three months.

Umbilical Cord: The cord that connects the baby to the placenta, providing nutrients and oxygen.

Ultrasound: A prenatal imaging technique that uses sound waves to visualize the baby and monitor its development.

Uterus: The muscular organ where the baby grows during pregnancy.

Vaccinations during Pregnancy: Immunizations recommended for pregnant women to protect both the mother and the baby.

Vacuum Extraction: A method used to assist in the delivery of the baby, using a suction cup attached to the baby's head.

Varicose Veins: Swollen, twisted veins often seen in the legs during pregnancy due to increased pressure on blood vessels.

Vernix: A waxy substance that covers the baby's skin in the womb, protecting it from amniotic fluid.

Vertex Position: When the baby's head is positioned downward, ready for a head-first delivery.

Water Breaking: The rupture of the amniotic sac, often referred to as "breaking the water," signaling the start of labor.

X-ray Safety during Pregnancy: Precautions to avoid exposure to X-rays during pregnancy, as they may harm the developing baby.

Checklists for Pregnancy, Labor, and Postpartum Preparation

Checklist for Pregnancy Preparation

- **Prenatal Vitamins**: Start taking prenatal vitamins with folic acid as soon as you plan to conceive.

- **Healthcare Provider**: Choose a healthcare provider, either an obstetrician or a midwife, to guide you through your pregnancy journey.

- **Prenatal Care Schedule**: Schedule regular prenatal check-ups and follow-ups with your chosen healthcare provider.

- **Healthy Diet**: Adopt a balanced and nutritious diet rich in fruits, vegetables, whole grains, and lean pro-teins.

- **Stay Hydrated**: Drink plenty of water to stay hy-drated throughout your pregnancy.

- **Exercise**: Engage in safe and moderate exercises approved by your healthcare provider.

- **Avoid Harmful Substances**: Stay away from alco-hol, smoking, and illegal drugs that can harm your baby.

- **Educate Yourself**: Read books, attend prenatal clas-ses, and seek reliable information about pregnancy and childbirth.

- **Create a Supportive Network**: Discuss your preg-nancy plans with family and friends for emotional support.
- **Financial Planning**: Assess your finances and plan for upcoming medical expenses and maternity leave.

Checklist for Labor Preparation

- **Birth Plan**: Create a birth plan outlining your pref-erences for labor and delivery.
- **Pack Your Hospital Bag**: Prepare essentials like comfortable clothing, toiletries, snacks, and items for the baby.
- **Comfort Measures**: Gather items that can help dur-ing labor, such as a birthing ball, heating pad, or re-laxation music.
- **Discuss Pain Relief Options**: Talk to your healthcare provider about pain relief choices like epidurals or natural techniques.
- **Learn Breathing Techniques**: Practice deep breath-ing and relaxation techniques to manage labor pains.
- **Transportation Plan**: Plan how you'll reach the hos-pital or birthing center when labor begins.
- **Emergency Contact List**: Keep a list of emergency contacts handy for you and your birth partner.

- **Birth Partner Support**: Discuss the role and respon-sibilities of your birth partner during labor.
- **Childcare Arrangements**: If you have older children, make arrangements for their care during your labor.
- **Reliable Communication**: Ensure you have a work-ing phone and charger to stay connected during la-bor.

Checklist for Postpartum Preparation

- **Postpartum Recovery Supplies**: Stock up on pads, nursing bras, and comfortable clothing for postpar-tum healing.
- **Postpartum Support**: Arrange for help from family or friends during the first few weeks after birth.
- **Breastfeeding Support**: Research local lactation consultants or attend breastfeeding classes.
- **Feeding Essentials**: Purchase breastfeeding or bot-tle-feeding supplies like pumps, bottles, and formula.
- **Sleeping Arrangements**: Set up a safe and cozy sleep space for the baby, such as a bassinet or crib.
- **Newborn Care Education**: Learn about baby care basics like diapering, bathing, and soothing tech-niques.
- **Meal Preparations**: Prepare and freeze nutritious meals for easy postpartum nourishment.
- **Postpartum Exercises**: Discuss safe exercises with your healthcare provider to aid postpartum recovery.
- **Self-Care**: Prioritize self-care, rest, and relaxation during the postpartum period.

- **Mental Health Support**: Plan to connect with sup-port groups or therapists for emotional well-being.

Remember, every pregnancy and childbirth experience is unique. Adapt these checklists to suit your individual needs and consult with your healthcare provider for personalized guidance throughout your journey.

Diet Plan during Pregnancy

Remember, individual nutritional needs can vary, so it's always best to consult a healthcare provider or registered dietitian for personalized guidance.

First Trimester Diet Plan

Meal	Nutrients	Description	Food Sources
Break-fast	Folate, Fiber, Protein	Folate prevents birth defects. Fiber aids digestion. Protein supports tissue growth.	Whole-grain toast, scrambled eggs, spinach, orange juice
Snack	Calcium, Protein	Calcium for bone development. Protein for energy.	Greek yogurt, almonds
Lunch	Iron, Vitamin C, Folate	Iron prevents anemia. Vitamin C enhances iron absorption. Folate supports fetal growth.	Grilled chicken salad with spinach, bell peppers, and citrus dressing

Meal	Nutrients	Description	Food Sources
Snack	Fiber, Vitamin A	Fiber aids digestion. Vitamin A supports vision.	Carrot sticks with hummus
Dinner	Omega-3 Fatty Acids, Protein	Omega-3s promote brain development. Protein supports tissue growth.	Baked salmon, quinoa, steamed broccoli
Snack	Calcium, Protein	Calcium for bone health. Protein for energy.	Cheese and whole-grain crackers

Second Trimester Diet Plan

Meal	Nutrients	Description	Food Sources
Break-fast	Calcium, Fiber, Protein	Calcium for bones. Fiber aids digestion. Protein supports tissue growth.	Whole-grain cereal with milk, sliced banana
Snack	Vitamin C, Protein	Vitamin C supports immunity. Protein for energy.	Orange slices, handful of nuts
Lunch	Iron, Folate, Vitamin K	Iron prevents anemia. Folate supports fetal growth. Vitamin K aids blood clotting.	Lentil soup, whole-grain roll, mixed greens
Snack	Fiber, Calcium	Fiber aids digestion. Calcium for bones.	Greek yogurt with berries

Meal	Nutrients	Description	Food Sources
Dinner	Protein, Vitamin D, Iron	Protein supports tissue growth. Vitamin D aids calcium absorption. Iron prevents anemia.	Grilled lean steak, sweet potato, sautéed spinach
Snack	Protein, Fiber	Protein for energy. Fiber aids digestion.	Cottage cheese with apple slices

Third Trimester Diet Plan

Meal	Nutrients	Description	Food Sources
Break-fast	Fiber, Pro-tein, Vitamin C	Fiber aids digestion. Protein supports tissue growth. Vitamin C enhances iron absorption.	Oatmeal with berries and nuts
Snack	Calcium, Pro-tein	Calcium for bones. Protein for energy.	Cheese and whole-grain crackers
Lunch	Folate, Iron, Omega-3 Fatty Acids	Folate supports fetal growth. Iron prevents anemia. Omega-3s promote brain development.	Grilled salmon salad with mixed greens, walnuts, and vinaigrette
Snack	Vitamin A, Fiber	Vitamin A supports vision. Fiber aids digestion.	Carrot sticks with hummus
Dinner	Protein, Calcium	Protein supports tissue growth. Calcium for bones.	Baked chicken

Meal	Nutrients	Description	Food Sources
			breast, quinoa, steamed vegetables
Snack	Protein, Fiber	Protein for energy. Fiber aids digestion.	Greek yogurt with granola

Key Nutrients and Their Sources

- **Folate**: Lentils, leafy greens, fortified cereals.
- **Iron**: Lean meats, beans, fortified grains.
- **Calcium**: Dairy products, fortified plant-based milk.
- **Vitamin C**: Citrus fruits, bell peppers, strawberries.
- **Omega-3 Fatty Acids**: Fatty fish (salmon, sardines), chia seeds.
- **Protein**: Lean meats, poultry, fish, beans, lentils.
- **Fiber**: Whole grains, fruits, vegetables, legumes.
- **Vitamin A**: Carrots, sweet potatoes, leafy greens.
- **Vitamin D**: Fatty fish, fortified dairy alternatives.

- **Vitamin K**: Leafy greens, broccoli, Brussels sprouts.

Remember to drink plenty of water and adjust portion sizes according to your appetite and needs. Always consult a healthcare provider before making significant changes to your diet during pregnancy.

Breastfeeding Tips for Mothers

Positioning

- Ensure a comfortable position for both you and your baby.
- Bring your baby close to your breast, aiming their nose at your nipple.

Latch On

- Wait for your baby to open their mouth wide before latching.
- Make sure their lips are flanged outward, covering more of the areola under the nipple.

Frequent Feeding

- Newborns feed often, about 8-12 times a day.
- Feed on demand, watching for hunger cues like rooting, sucking motions, or fussiness.

Empty One Breast

- Allow your baby to feed on one breast until they naturally release.
- This ensures they get the nutrient-rich hind-milk that comes after the initial foremilk.

Burping

- Gently burp your baby midway through and after feeding.

- Support their head and back, patting or rub-
  bing their back softly.

Hydration and Nutrition

- Drink plenty of fluids to stay hydrated.
- Eat a balanced diet rich in fruits, vegetables,
  whole grains, and lean proteins.

Comfortable Environment

- Choose a quiet, cozy spot for nursing to mini-
  mize distractions.
- Have pillows to support your back and arms.

Breast Care

- Keep nipples clean and dry.
- Apply lanolin cream or breast milk to soothe
  sore nipples.

Rest and Self-Care

- Rest when your baby sleeps.
- Take care of yourself – a well-rested mom
  produces more milk.

Pumping and Storing

- If needed, pump to build a milk supply or to
  have milk on hand when you're away.
- Store breast milk in clean, labeled containers
  in the *fridge or freezer.*

Seeking Help

- If you're experiencing pain or difficulties, consult a lactation consultant or a healthcare provider.
- Don't hesitate to ask for advice or support from experienced moms or support groups.

Trust Your Instincts

- Every baby and breastfeeding journey is unique.
- Trust yourself and your baby's cues – you're both learning together.

Remember, breastfeeding can be a learning process for both you and your baby. Be patient and kind to yourself as you navigate this new experience.